The Super Easy Ketogenic Recipe Guide

Quick and Easy Ketogenic Recipes to Boost Your Diet and Improve Your Body

Lauren Loose

© **Copyright 2021 - All rights reserved.**

The content contained within this book may not be reproduced, duplicated or transmitted without direct written permission from the author or the publisher.

Under no circumstances will any blame or legal responsibility be held against the publisher, or author, for any damages, reparation, or monetary loss due to the information contained within this book. Either directly or indirectly.

Legal Notice:

This book is copyright protected. This book is only for personal use. You cannot amend, distribute, sell, use, quote or paraphrase any part, or the content within this book, without the consent of the author or publisher.

Disclaimer Notice:

Please note the information contained within this document is for educational and entertainment purposes only. All effort has been executed to present accurate, up to date, and reliable, complete information. No warranties of any kind are declared or implied. Readers acknowledge that the author is not engaging in the rendering of legal, financial, medical or professional advice. The content within this book has been derived from various sources. Please consult a licensed professional before attempting any techniques outlined in this book.

By reading this document, the reader agrees that under no circumstances is the author responsible for any losses, direct or indirect, which are incurred as a result of the use of information contained within this document, including, but not limited to, — errors, omissions, or inaccuracies.

Contents

Beef and Broccoli Stir-Fry 8
Parmesan-Crusted Halibut with Asparagus 10
Hearty Beef and Bacon Casserole 12
Sesame Wings with Cauliflower 14
Fried Coconut Shrimp   with Asparagus 16
Coconut Chicken Curry with Cauliflower Rice 18
Grilled Whole Chicken 20
Grilled Chicken Breast 22
Glazed Chicken Thighs 23
Bacon-Wrapped Chicken Breasts 25
Chicken Parmigiana 27
Bacon Burger Stir Fry 29
Bacon Cheeseburger 30
Cauliflower Mac & Cheese 31
Mushroom &   Cauliflower Risotto 32
Pita Pizza 33
Skillet Cabbage Tacos 34
Taco Casserole 35
Creamy Chicken Salad 36
Spicy Ketogenic Chicken Wings 37
Cilantro and Lime   Creamed Chicken 38
Cheesy Ham Quiche 40
Loaded Cauliflower Rice 41
Creamy Garlic Chicken 42
Chinese Pork Bowl 44
Relatively Flavored Gratin 45

Low Carb Crack Slaw Egg Roll 47

Low Carb Beef Stir Fry 49

Pesto Chicken and Veggies 50

Crispy Peanut Tofu and Cauliflower Rice Stir-Fry 52

Ketogenic Fried Chicken 54

Meatballs in Mushroom Sauce 56

Roasted Chicken 58

Lemony Chicken Drumsticks 60

Stuffed Chicken Breasts 61

Chicken with Capers Sauce 63

Lemony Chicken Thighs 65

Bacon-Wrapped Turkey Breast 67

Turkey Meatloaf 68

Herbed Beef Tenderloin 70

Steak with Cheese Sauce 72

Steak with Pesto 74

Herbed Lamb Chops 75

Stuffed Leg of Lamb 76

Grilled Pork Chops 78

Pork Chops in Cream Sauce 79

Garlicky Prime Rib Roast 81

Beef Wellington 82

Beef with Mushroom Sauce 84

Herbed Rack of Lamb 86

Roasted Leg of Lamb 88

Baked lamb ribs macadamia with tomato salsa 90

Grilled Garlic Butter Shrimp 92

Tomato Chili Chicken Tender with Fresh Basils 94
Pork crack slaw 96
Ketogenic lasagna 98
Easy meal prep chicken soup 101
Ketogenic burger 103
Calamari mayo with cauliflower broccoli salad 105
Ketogenic strawberry rice 107

Beef and Broccoli Stir-Fry

Preparation Time: 20 minutes

Cooking Time: 15 minutes

Servings: 4

Ingredients:

- ¼ cup soy sauce
- 1 tablespoon sesame oil
- 1 teaspoon garlic chili paste
- 1-pound beef sirloin
- 2 tablespoons almond flour
- 2 tablespoons coconut oil
- 2 cups chopped broccoli florets
- 1 tablespoon grated ginger
- 3 cloves garlic, minced

Directions:

1. In a small bowl, whisk the soy sauce, sesame oil, and chili paste together. In a plastic freezer bag, slice the beef and mix with the almond flour. Pour in the sauce and toss to coat for 20 minutes, then let rest.
2. Heat up the oil over medium to high heat in a large skillet. In the pan, add the beef and sauce and cook until the beef is browned.

3. Move the beef to the skillet sides, then add the broccoli, ginger, and garlic. Sauté until tender-crisp broccoli, then throw it all together and serve hot.

Nutrition:

350 Calories

19g Fats

37g Protein

6g Carbohydrates

Parmesan-Crusted Halibut with Asparagus

Preparation Time: 10 minutes

Cooking Time: 15 minutes

Servings: 4

Ingredients:

- 2 tablespoons olive oil
- ¼ cup butter, softened
- Salt and pepper
- ¼ cup grated Parmesan
- 1-pound asparagus, trimmed
- 2 tablespoons almond flour
- 4 (6-ounce) boneless halibut fillets
- 1 teaspoon garlic powder

Directions:

1. Preheat the oven to 400 F and line a foil-based baking sheet. Throw the asparagus in olive oil and scatter over the baking sheet.
2. In a blender, add the butter, Parmesan cheese, almond flour, garlic powder, salt and pepper, and mix until smooth. Place the fillets with the asparagus on the baking sheet, and spoon the Parmesan over the eggs.
3. Bake for 10 to 12 minutes, then broil until browned for 2 to 3 minutes.

Nutrition:

415 Calories

26g Fats

42g Protein

3g Carbohydrates

Hearty Beef and Bacon Casserole

Preparation Time: 25 minutes

Cooking Time: 30 minutes

Servings: 8

Ingredients:

- 8 slices uncooked bacon
- 1 medium head cauliflower, chopped
- ¼ cup canned coconut milk
- Salt and pepper
- 2 pounds ground beef (80% lean)
- 8 ounces mushrooms, sliced
- 1 large yellow onion, chopped
- 2 cloves garlic, minced

Directions:

1. Preheat to 375 F on the oven. Cook the bacon in a skillet until crispy, then drain and chop on paper towels.
2. Bring to boil a pot of salted water, then add the cauliflower. Boil until tender for 6 to 8 minutes then drain and add the coconut milk to a food processor. Mix until smooth, then sprinkle with salt and pepper.
3. Cook the beef until browned in a pan, then wash the fat away. Remove the mushrooms,

onion, and garlic, then move to a baking platter. Place on top of the cauliflower mixture and bake for 30 minutes. Broil for 5 minutes on high heat, then sprinkle with bacon to serve.

Nutrition:

410 Calories

25g Fats

37g Protein

6g Carbohydrates

Sesame Wings with Cauliflower

Preparation Time: 5 minutes

Cooking Time: 30 minutes

Servings: 4

Ingredients:

- 2 ½ tablespoons soy sauce
- 2 tablespoons sesame oil
- 1 ½ teaspoons balsamic vinegar
- 1 teaspoon minced garlic
- 1 teaspoon grated ginger
- Salt
- 1-pound chicken wing, the wings itself
- 2 cups cauliflower florets

Directions:

1. In a freezer bag, mix the soy sauce, sesame oil, balsamic vinegar, garlic, ginger, and salt, then add the chicken wings. Coat flip, then chill for 2 to 3 hours.
2. Preheat the oven to 400 F and line a foil-based baking sheet. Spread the wings along with the cauliflower onto the baking sheet. Bake for 35 minutes, then sprinkle on to serve with sesame seeds.

Nutrition:

400 Calories

15g Fats

5g Protein

3g Carbohydrates

Fried Coconut Shrimp with Asparagus

Preparation Time: 15 minutes

Cooking Time: 10 minutes

Servings: 6

Ingredients:

- 1 ½ cups shredded unsweetened coconut
- 2 large eggs
- Salt and pepper
- 1 ½ pounds large shrimp, peeled and deveined
- ½ cup canned coconut milk
- 1-pound asparagus, cut into 2-inch pieces

Directions:

1. Pour the coconut onto a shallow platter. Beat the eggs in a bowl with a little salt and pepper. Dip the shrimp into the egg first, then dredge with coconut.
2. Heat up coconut oil over medium-high heat in a large skillet. Add the shrimp and fry over each side for 1 to 2 minutes until browned.
3. Remove the paper towels from the shrimp and heat the skillet again. Remove the asparagus and sauté to tender-crisp with salt and pepper, then serve with the shrimp.

Nutrition:

535 Calories

38g Fats

16g Protein

3g Carbohydrates

Coconut Chicken Curry with Cauliflower Rice

Preparation time: 15 minutes

Cooking time: 30 minutes

Servings: 6

Ingredients:

- 1 tablespoon olive oil
- 1 medium yellow onion, chopped
- 1 ½ pounds boneless chicken thighs, chopped
- Salt and pepper
- 1 (14-ounce) can coconut milk
- 1 tablespoon curry powder
- 1 ¼ teaspoon ground turmeric
- 3 cups riced cauliflower

Directions:

1. Heat the oil over medium heat, in a large skillet. Add the onions, and cook for about 5 minutes, until translucent.
2. Stir in the chicken and season with salt and pepper-cook for 6 to 8 minutes, stirring frequently until all sides are browned. Pour the coconut milk into the pan, then whisk in the curry and turmeric powder.
3. Simmer until hot and bubbling, for 15 to 20 minutes. Meanwhile, steam the cauliflower rice

until tender with a few tablespoons of water. Serve the cauliflower rice over the curry.

Nutrition:

430 Calories

29g Fats

9g Protein

3g Carbohydrates

Grilled Whole Chicken

Preparation Time: 20 minutes

Cooking Time: 20 minutes

Servings: 6

Ingredients

- ¼ cup butter
- 2 tablespoons lemon juice
- 2 teaspoons fresh lemon zest
- 1 teaspoon dried oregano
- 2 teaspoons paprika
- 1 teaspoon onion powder
- 1 teaspoon garlic powder
- Salt and ground black pepper
- 1 (4-pound) grass-fed whole chicken

Directions:

1. Preheat the grill to medium heat. Grease the grill grate. Place onto a large cutting board, breast-side down. Mix butter, lemon juice, lemon zest, oregano, spices, salt, and black pepper.
2. Cut both sides of backbone. Remove the backbone. Flip and open. Firmly press breast to flatten.

3. Coat the whole chicken with the oil mixture. Grill for 20 minutes.
4. Remove from the grill and set aside for 10 minutes.

Nutrition:

532 Calories

17g Fat

0.5g Fiber

Grilled Chicken Breast

Preparation Time: 15 minutes

Cooking Time: 14 minutes

Servings: 4

Ingredients

- ¼ cup balsamic vinegar
- 2 tablespoons olive oil
- 1½ teaspoons lemon juice
- ½ teaspoon lemon-pepper seasoning
- 4 (6-ounce) grass-fed chicken breast halves

Directions:

1. Blend vinegar, oil, lemon juice, and seasoning. Coat chicken breasts with the mixture. Marinate for 30 minutes.
2. Preheat and grease the grill to medium heat. Place the chicken breasts onto the grill and cover.
3. Cook for 7 minutes. Serve.

Nutrition:

258 Calories

11.3g Fat

0.1g Fiber

Glazed Chicken Thighs

Preparation Time: 15 minutes

Cooking Time: 35 minutes

Servings: 8

Ingredients

- ½ cup balsamic vinegar
- 1/3 cup low-sodium soy sauce
- 3 tablespoons Yukon syrup
- 4 tablespoons olive oil
- 3 tablespoons chili sauce
- 2 tablespoons garlic
- Salt and black pepper
- 8 (6-ounce) grass-fed chicken thighs

Directions:

1. Mix all ingredients (except chicken thighs and sesame seeds). Mix half of marinade and chicken thighs. Seal and shake well.
2. Chill for 1 hour. Chill remaining marinade. Preheat oven to 425ºF.
3. Mix reserved marinade over medium heat and boil. Cook for 5 minutes. Remove and set aside.
4. Remove from the bag and discard excess marinade. Arrange chicken thighs into a 9x13-

inch baking dish in a single layer and coat with cooked marinade.

5. Bake for 30 minutes. Serve.

Nutrition:

406 Calories

19.6g Fat

0.1g Fiber

Bacon-Wrapped Chicken Breasts

Preparation Time: 15 minutes

Cooking Time: 33 minutes

Servings: 4

Ingredients

Chicken Marinade

- 3 tablespoons balsamic vinegar
- 3 tablespoons olive oil
- 2 tablespoons water
- 1 garlic clove
- 1 teaspoon dried Italian seasoning
- ½ teaspoon dried rosemary
- 4 (6-ounce) grass-fed chicken breasts

Stuffing

- 16 fresh basil leaves
- 1 large fresh tomato
- 4 provolone cheese slices
- 8 bacon slices
- ¼ cup Parmesan cheese

Directions:
1. For marinade:
    a. Mix all ingredients (except chicken).
2. For chicken

3. Chop chicken breast horizontally, without cutting all the way through.
4. Repeat with the remaining chicken breasts. Coat with marinade. Chill 30 minutes.
5. Preheat your oven to 500ºF. Grease baking dish.
6. Place 4 basil leaves onto the bottom half of a chicken breast. Followed by 3 tomato slices and 1 provolone cheese slice. Fold the top half over filling.
7. Wrap the breast with 3 bacon slices. Repeat. Situate into the prepared baking dish in a single layer.
8. Bake for 30 minutes. Remove and sprinkle with Parmesan cheese evenly. Bake for 3 minutes more.

Nutrition:

633 Calories

36g Fat

0.3g Fiber

Chicken Parmigiana

Preparation Time: 15 minutes

Cooking Time: 26 minutes

Servings: 5

Ingredients

- 5 (6-ounce) grass-fed chicken breasts
- 1 large organic egg
- ½ cup superfine almond flour
- ¼ cup Parmesan cheese,
- ½ teaspoon dried parsley
- ½ teaspoon paprika
- ½ teaspoon garlic powder
- 1 cup sugar-free tomato sauce
- 5 ounces mozzarella cheese
- 2 tablespoons fresh parsley

Directions:

1. Preheat your oven to 375ºF. Wrap 1 chicken breast in parchment paper. Pound the chicken breast into ½-inch thickness
2. Repeat with the rest. Put the beaten egg. Mix almond flour, Parmesan, parsley, spices, salt, and black pepper in another dish.

3. Dip it into the whipped egg and coat with the flour mixture. Heat the oil over medium-high heat and fry for 3 minutes.
4. Dry chicken breasts. Spread at bottom of a casserole dish ½ cup of tomato sauce. Arrange the chicken breasts over marinara sauce in a single layer.
5. Drizzle with the remaining tomato sauce, mozzarella cheese slices. Bake for 20 minutes. Garnish with parsley. Serve

Nutrition:

458 Calories

25.4g Fat

7.9g Carbs

Bacon Burger Stir Fry

Preparation Time: 10 minutes

Cooking Time: 20 minutes

Servings: 10

Ingredients:
- 1 lb. Ground beef
- 1 lb. Bacon
- 1 Small onion
- 3 garlic cloves
- 1 Cabbage

Directions:
1. Dice the bacon and onion. Mix the beef and bacon in a wok.
2. Mince the onion and garlic. Toss both into the hot grease. Slice and toss in the cabbage and stir-fry. Mix in the meat and season.

Nutrition:

32g Protein

22g Fats

357 Calories

Bacon Cheeseburger

Preparation Time: 15 minutes

Cooking Time: 30 minutes

Servings: 12

Ingredients:

- 16 oz. Low-sodium bacon
- 3 lb. Ground beef
- 2 Eggs
- ½ Medium onion
- 8 oz. cheddar cheese

Directions:

1. Fry the bacon and chop it to bits. Shred the cheese and dice the onion. Mix the mixture with the beef and whisked eggs.
2. Grill 24 burger if desired.

Nutrition:

27g Protein

41g Fats

489 Calories

Cauliflower Mac & Cheese

Preparation Time: 15 minutes

Cooking Time: 20 minutes

Servings: 4

Ingredients:

- 1 Cauliflower
- 3 tbsp. Butter
- ¼ cup unsweetened almond milk
- ¼ cup Heavy cream
- 1 cup Cheddar cheese

Directions:

1. Slice the cauliflower into small florets. Shred the cheese. Prepare the oven to 450º Fahrenheit. Wrap baking pan with foil.
2. Melt two tablespoons butter. Mix the florets, butter, salt, and pepper. Roast the cauliflower on the baking pan for 15 minutes.
3. Warm rest of the butter, milk, heavy cream, and cheese in the microwave. Pour the cheese and serve.

Nutrition:

11g Protein

23g Fats

294 Calories

Mushroom & Cauliflower Risotto

Preparation Time: 5 minutes

Cooking Time: 10 minutes

Servings: 4

Ingredients:

- 1 cauliflower
- 1 cup Vegetable stock
- 9 oz. mushrooms
- 2 tbsp. Butter
- 1 cup Coconut cream

Directions:

1. Pour the stock in a saucepan. Boil and set aside. Prepare a skillet with butter and sauté the mushrooms.
2. Grate and stir in the cauliflower and stock. Simmer and add the cream. Serve.

Nutrition:

1g Protein

17g Fats

186 Calories

Pita Pizza

Preparation Time: 15 minutes

Cooking Time: 10 minutes

Servings: 2

Ingredients:

- ½ cup Marinara sauce
- 1 Low-carb pita
- 2 oz. Cheddar cheese
- 14 Pepperoni slices
- 1 oz. Roasted red peppers

Directions:

1. Set oven to 450º Fahrenheit.
2. Slice the pita in half and place onto a foil-lined baking tray. Rub with a bit of oil and toast for 2 minutes.
3. Pour the sauce over the bread. Sprinkle using the cheese and other toppings. Bake for 5 minutes.

Nutrition:

13g Protein

19g Fats

250 Calories

Skillet Cabbage Tacos

Preparation Time: 10 minutes

Cooking Time: 15 minutes

Servings: 4

Ingredients:

- 1 lb. Ground beef
- ½ cup Salsa
- 2 cups cabbage
- 2 tsp. Chili powder
- ¾ cup cheese

Directions:

1. Brown the beef and drain the fat. Pour in the salsa, cabbage, and seasoning.
2. Cover and lower the heat. Simmer 12 minutes using the medium heat.
3. Once softened, remove it from the heat and mix in the cheese.
4. Top with green onions.

Nutrition:

30g Protein

21g Fats

325 Calories

Taco Casserole

Preparation Time: 10 minutes

Cooking Time: 20 minutes

Servings: 8

Ingredients:

- 2 lbs. Ground beef
- 2 tbsp. Taco seasoning
- 8 oz. cheddar cheese
- 1 cup Salsa
- 16 oz. Cottage cheese

Directions:

1. Heat the oven to 400° Fahrenheit.
2. Combine the taco seasoning and ground meat in a casserole dish. Bake for 20 minutes.
3. Combine the salsa and both kinds of cheese. Set aside.
4. Drain away the cooking juices from the meat.
5. Mash the meat into small pieces.
6. Sprinkle with cheese. Bake in the oven for 20.

Nutrition:

45g Protein

18g Fats

367 Calories

Creamy Chicken Salad

Preparation Time: 10 minutes

Cooking Time: 30 minutes

Servings: 4

Ingredients:

- 1 lb. Chicken Breast
- 2 Avocados
- 2 Garlic Cloves
- 3 tbsp. Lime Juice
- 1/3 cup Onion
- 1 Jalapeno Pepper
- 1 tbsp. Cilantro

Directions

1. Set oven to 400 F. Line cooking sheet with foil. Layer the chicken breast up with some olive oil before seasoning.
2. Situate onto cooking sheet and put into the oven for 20 minutes. Let it cool and shred. Combine everything into a bowl and mash the avocado. Season well!

Nutrition:

20g Fats

4g Carbohydrates

25g Protein

Spicy Ketogenic Chicken Wings

Preparation Time: 20 Minutes

Cooking Time: 30 minutes

Servings: 4

Ingredients:

- 2 lbs. Chicken Wings
- 1 tsp. Cajun Spice
- 2 tsp. Smoked Paprika
- ½ tsp. Turmeric
- 2 tsp. Baking Powder

Directions:

1. Prep the stove to 400 F. Dry chicken wings with a paper towel.
2. Mix all of the seasonings along with the baking powder. Toss the chicken wings in and coat evenly. Put on a wire rack that is placed over your baking tray.
3. Cook for 30 minutes. Pull out from the oven and flip to bake the other side for 30 minutes.
4. Take it out and set aside. Serve.

Nutrition:

7g Fats

1g Carbohydrates

60g Proteins

Cilantro and Lime Creamed Chicken

Preparation Time: 10 Minutes

Cooking Time: 20 minutes

Servings: 4

Ingredients:

- 4 Chicken Breast
- 1 tsp. Red Pepper Flakes
- 1 tbsp. Cilantro
- 2 tbsp. Lime Juice
- 1 cup Chicken Broth
- ¼ cup Onion
- 1 tbsp. Olive Oil
- ½ cup Heavy Cream

Directions:

1. Preheat skillet and place it over a moderate temperature. Season the chicken breast. Throw into the skillet and cook for 8 minutes on each side. Set aside
2. Stir in the onion and cook them for a minute then mix in cilantro, pepper flakes, lime juice, and the chicken broth.

3. Boil for 10 minutes. Whisk in your heavy cream and add in the chicken to coat.

Nutrition:

20g Fats

6g Carbohydrates

30g Proteins

Cheesy Ham Quiche

Preparation Time: 10 minutes

Cooking Time: 30 minutes

Servings: 6

Ingredients:

- 8 Eggs
- 1 cup Zucchini
- ½ cup heavy Cream
- 1 cup Ham
- 1 tsp. Mustard

Directions:

1. Prep stove to 375 and get pie plate for your quiche. Shred the zucchini.
2. Once done, drain. Place the zucchini into your pie plate along with the cooked ham pieces and cheese. Whisk the seasonings, cream, and eggs. Pour on top then cook for 40 minutes.
3. If the quiche is cooked to your liking, take the dish from the oven and allow it to chill slightly before slicing.

Nutrition:

25g Fats

2g Carbohydrates

20g Proteins

Loaded Cauliflower Rice

Preparation Time: 10 minutes

Cooking Time: 20 minutes

Servings: 4

Ingredients:

- 1 Cauliflower
- 1 cup Cheddar Cheese
- 1 lb. Bacon
- ½ cup Chives

Directions:

1. Rice your cauliflower. You can choose to do this by hand. Cook the bacon in a grilling pan over a medium heat.
2. Place your cauliflower rice into a microwave-safe bowl and sprinkle your shredded cheese over the top.
3. Place bowl into the microwave for a minute and allow for the rice to cook through and the cheese to melt. Top with your bacon pieces and season to your liking.

Nutrition:

10g Fats

5g Carbohydrates

5g Proteins

Creamy Garlic Chicken

Preparation Time: 5 minutes

Cooking Time: 15 minutes

Servings: 4

Ingredients:
- 4 chicken breasts
- 1 tsp. garlic powder
- 1 tsp. paprika
- 2 tbsp. butter
- 1 tsp. salt
- 1 cup heavy cream
- ½ cup sun-dried tomatoes
- 2 cloves garlic
- 1 cup spinach

Directions:
1. Blend the paprika, garlic powder, and salt and rub both sides of the chicken.
2. Melt the butter in a frying pan over medium heat. Fry chicken for 5 minutes each side. Set aside.
3. Whisk the heavy cream, sun-dried tomatoes, and garlic. Cook for 2 minutes. Sauté spinach for additional 3 minutes. Place chicken back to the pan and cover with the sauce.

Nutrition:

12g Carbohydrates

26g Fat

4g Protein

Chinese Pork Bowl

Preparation Time: 5 minutes

Cooking Time: 15 minutes

Servings: 4

Ingredients:

- 1¼ pounds pork belly
- 2 Tbsp. tamari soy sauce
- 1 Tbsp. rice vinegar
- 2 cloves garlic
- 3 oz. butter
- 1-pound Brussels sprouts
- ½ leek

Directions:

1. Fry the pork over medium-high heat.
2. Combine the garlic cloves, butter, and Brussels sprouts. Add in to the pan and cook.
3. Drizzle soy sauce and rice vinegar together and pour into the pan. Season.
4. Top with chopped leek.

Nutrition:

7g Carbohydrates

97g Protein

993 Calories

Relatively Flavored Gratin

Preparation Time: 15 minutes

Cooking Time: 46 minutes

Servings: 8

Ingredients:

- ½ C. heavy whipping cream
- 2 tbsp. butter
- ½ tsp. garlic powder
- ¼ tsp. xanthan gum
- 4 C. zucchini
- 1 small yellow onion
- 1½ C. pepper jack cheese

Directions:

1. Prepare oven to 375 0 F and grease a 9×9-inch baking dish. In a microwave-safe dish, mix heavy whipping cream, butter, garlic powder, and xanthan gum and melt 1 minute.
2. Arrange 1/3 of zucchini and onion slices at the bottom and season and ½ C. of pepper jack cheese. Repeat the layers twice. Spread the cream mixture on top evenly. Bake for 45 minutes. Remove the baking dish from oven and set aside.

Nutrition:

140 Calories

3.9g Carbohydrates

5.5g Protein

Low Carb Crack Slaw Egg Roll

Preparation time: 10 minutes

Cooking Time: 20 minutes

Serving: 2

Ingredients:
- 1 lb. ground beef
- 4 cups shredded coleslaw mix
- 1 tbsp. avocado oil
- 1 tsp. sea salt
- ¼ tsp. black pepper
- 4 cloves garlic, minced
- 3 tbsp. fresh ginger, grated
- ¼ cup coconut amines
- 2 tsp. toasted sesame oil
- ¼ cup green onions

Directions:
1. Cook avocado oil over medium-high heat. Cook the garlic.
2. Cook ground beef for 10 minutes. Season well.
3. Once cooked, you can lower the heat and add the coleslaw mix and the coconut amines. Stir for 5 minutes.
4. Garnish green onions and the toasted sesame oil.

Nutrition:

104 calories

5g fat

18g protein

Low Carb Beef Stir Fry

Preparation Time: 10 minutes

Cooking Time: 25 minutes

Serving: 3

Ingredients:

- ½ cup zucchini
- ¼ cup organic broccoli florets
- 1 bunch baby bok choy
- 2 tbsp. avocado oil
- 2 tsp. coconut amines
- 1 small ginger
- 8 oz. skirt steak

Directions:

1. Heat the pan and add 1 tbsp. oil. Sear steak on high heat for 2 minutes per side.
2. Set to medium heat and cook the broccoli, ginger, ghee, and coconut amines.
3. Cook the book choy for another minute
4. Mix in zucchini and cook.

Nutrition:

104 calories

6g fat

31g protein

Pesto Chicken and Veggies

Preparation Time: 10 minutes

Cooking Time: 35 minutes

Serving: 3

Ingredients:

- 2 tbsp. olive oil
- 1 cup cherry tomatoes
- ¼ cup basil pesto
- 1/3 cup sun-dried tomatoes
- 1-pound chicken thigh
- 1-pound asparagus

Directions:

1. Preheat two tablespoons of olive oil and sliced chicken on medium heat. Season and add ½ cup of the sun-dried tomatoes.
2. Cook well. Spoon out the chicken and tomatoes and put them in a separate container.
3. Place the asparagus in same skillet and pour in the pesto. Put heat on medium and add the remaining sun-dried tomatoes. Cook for 10 minutes. Put it on a separate plate.
4. Position the chicken back in the pan and pour in pesto. Stir over medium heat for 2 minutes.

Nutrition:

104 calories

8g fat

26g protein

Crispy Peanut Tofu and Cauliflower Rice Stir-Fry

Preparation Time: 10 minutes

Cooking Time: 80 minutes

Serving: 4

Ingredients:

- 12 oz. tofu
- 1 tbsp. sesame oil
- 2 cloves garlic
- 1 small cauliflower head

For the sauce:

- 1 ½ tbsp. sesame oil
- ½ tsp. chili garlic sauce
- 2 ½ tbsp. peanut butter
- ¼ cup low sodium soy sauce
- ½ cup light brown sugar

Directions:

1. Strain tofu for 90 minutes.
2. Preheat the oven to 400 degrees Fahrenheit. Cube the tofu, and prepare your baking sheet.
3. Bake for 25 minutes and allow it to cool.
4. Combine the sauce ingredients.
5. Put the tofu in the sauce and coat the tofu thoroughly. Leave it for 15 minutes.
6. Shred the cauliflower into rice- size bits.

7. Situate skillet on medium heat. Cook veggies on a bit of sesame oil and soy sauce. Set aside.
8. Put tofu on the pan. Stir frequently. Set aside.
9. Steam your cauliflower rice for 8 minutes. Stir some sauce.
10. Mix ingredients together. Mix cauliflower rice with the veggies and tofu. Serve.

Nutrition:

107 calories

9g fat

30g protein

Ketogenic Fried Chicken

Preparation Time: 10 minutes

Cooking Time: 45 minutes

Serving: 4

Ingredients:
- 4 chicken thighs
- Frying oil
- 2 large eggs
- 2 tbsp. heavy whipping cream

For the breading:
- 2/3 cup parmesan cheese
- 2/3 cup almond flour
- 1 tsp. salt
- ½ tsp. black pepper
- ½ tsp. cayenne
- ½ tsp. paprika

Directions:
1. Beat together the eggs and heavy cream.
2. Mix all the breading ingredients. Set aside.
3. Cut the chicken thigh into 3 even pieces and pat dry with paper towel.

4. Dip the chicken in the bread first before dipping it in the egg wash and then finally, dipping it in the breading again.
5. Fill 2 inches of oil in a pot and preheat at 350 degrees Fahrenheit. Gradually lower the heat.
6. Put the coated chicken in your hot oil. Fry for 5 minutes.
7. Strain cooked chicken.
8. Try not to overcrowd the pan. Serve.

Nutrition:

104 calories

5g fat

29g protein

Meatballs in Mushroom Sauce

Preparation Time: 20 minutes

Cooking Time: 15 minutes

Servings: 6

Ingredients

Meatballs

- 2 pounds ground turkey
- 2 medium eggs
- 1 onion
- 2 garlic cloves
- Salt and black pepper

Mushroom Sauce

- 1 tablespoon butter
- 3 ounces fresh mushrooms
- 3½ ounces cream cheese
- 1 cup homemade chicken broth
- Salt and black pepper
- 1 tablespoon parsley

Directions:

a. Preheat the oven to 350ºF. Prep baking sheet using parchment paper.

2. For meatballs:

3. Mix all the ingredients and roll into ball. Arrange in one layer onto the prepared baking sheet. Bake for 15 minutes.
4. For mushroom sauce:
5. Preheat the oil over medium heat and cook the mushrooms for 6 minutes. Cook cream cheese and broth for 4 minutes. Season and remove from the heat.
6. Topped with mushroom sauce. Garnish with parsley and serve.

Nutrition:

409 Calories

3.3g Carbs

46g Protein

Roasted Chicken

Preparation Time: 15 minutes

Cooking Time: 70 minutes

Servings: 5

Ingredients

- 3 tablespoons olive oil
- 3 garlic cloves
- 2 teaspoons lime zest
- 2 teaspoons dried rosemary
- Salt and black pepper
- 1 (3-pounds) grass-fed frying chicken

Directions:

1. Mix all the ingredients except the chicken. Coat chicken with mixture. Marinate overnight.
2. Preheat the oven to 425ºF. Put the chicken in pan then coat with marinade.
3. Knot the legs and tuck the wings back under. Roast for 10 minutes.
4. Set to 350ºF and roast for 1½ hours. Remove from oven and set aside 10 minutes.
5. Cut the chicken and serve.

Nutrition:

594 Calories

1g Total Carbs

78.9g Protein

Lemony Chicken Drumsticks

Preparation Time: 15 minutes

Cooking Time: 40 minutes

Servings: 6

Ingredients

- 3 pounds grass-fed chicken drumsticks
- ½ cup butter
- ¼ cup lemon juice
- 2 teaspoons garlic
- 2 teaspoons Italian seasoning
- Salt and ground white pepper

Directions:

1. Mix butter, lemon juice, garlic, Italian seasoning, salt, and black pepper. Coat chicken drumsticks with marinade.
2. Cover and refrigerate for 5 hours. Preheat the oven to 400ºF. Grease a large baking sheet.
3. Place in prepared baking sheet in a single layer. Bake for 40 minutes. Serve hot

Nutrition:

528 Calories

28.8g Fat

62.7g Protein

Stuffed Chicken Breasts

Preparation Time: 15 minutes

Cooking Time: 30 minutes

Servings: 4

Ingredients

- 1 teaspoon paprika
- ¼ teaspoon onion powder
- ¼ teaspoon garlic powder
- Salt
- 4 grass-fed chicken breasts
- 1 tablespoon olive oil
- 4 ounces cream cheese
- ¼ cup Parmesan cheese
- 2 tablespoons mayonnaise
- 1½ cups fresh spinach
- 1 teaspoon garlic
- ½ teaspoon red pepper flakes

Directions:

1. Preheat the oven to 375ºF. Mix spices and salt. Place chicken breasts in cutting board. Drizzle with oil.
2. Rub with spice mixture. Chop pocket into the side of each chicken breast. Mix cream cheese,

Parmesan, mayonnaise, spinach, garlic, red pepper, and ½ teaspoon salt.
3. Stuff with spinach mixture. Transfer into a 9x13-inch baking dish. Bake for 30 minutes. Serve.

Nutrition

468 Calories

30.2g Fat

45.7g Protein

Chicken with Capers Sauce

Preparation Time: 15 minutes

Cooking Time: 22 minutes

Servings: 2

Ingredients

- 2 (5½-ounces) grass-fed boneless
- Salt and black pepper
- 1/3 cup almond flour
- 2 tablespoons Parmesan cheese
- ½ teaspoon garlic powder
- 4 tablespoons olive oil
- 1 tablespoon garlic
- 3 tablespoons capers
- ¼ teaspoon red pepper flakes
- 3–4 tablespoons lemon juice
- 1 cup homemade chicken broth
- 1/3 cup heavy cream

Directions:

1. Season the chicken breasts. Mix flour, parmesan cheese and garlic powder.
2. Cover chicken breasts with the flour mixture. Preheat the oil in wok over medium-high heat and cook for 5 minutes per side.

3. Cover chicken thighs with foil. Pull out oil from the wok, leaving 1 tablespoon inside. Mix capers, garlic, red pepper flakes, lemon juice, and broth.
4. Mix the capers mixture over medium heat. Cook for 10 minutes. Stir in the heavy cream.
5. Return wok over medium heat and cook for 1 minute. Stir in the cooked chicken and remove from the heat. Serve.

Nutrition

783 Calories

59.4g Fat

50.7g Protein

Lemony Chicken Thighs

Preparation Time: 10 minutes

Cooking Time: 16 minutes

Servings: 4

Ingredients

- 2 tablespoons olive oil
- 1 tablespoon lemon juice
- 1 tablespoon lemon zest
- 2 teaspoons dried oregano
- 1 teaspoon dried thyme
- Salt and black pepper
- 1½ pounds grass-fed bone-in chicken thighs

Directions:

1. Preheat the oven to 420ºF. Mix 1 tablespoon of the oil, lemon juice, lemon zest, dried herbs, salt, and black pepper.
2. Coat chicken thighs with mixture. Marinate for 20 minutes. In oven-proof wok, heat oil over medium-high heat and sear chicken thighs for 3 minutes per side.
3. Situate into the oven and bake for 10 minutes. Serve.

Nutrition

388 Calories

19.7g Fat
49.4g Protein

Bacon-Wrapped Turkey Breast

Preparation Time: 10 minutes

Cooking Time: 1 hour

Servings: 2

Ingredients

- ¾ pound turkey breast
- ½ teaspoons dried rosemary
- ½ teaspoons dried thyme
- ½ teaspoons dried sage
- 6 large bacon slices

Directions:

1. Preheat the oven to 350°F. Ready baking sheet with a parchment paper. Sprinkle with herbs.
2. Wrap the bacon slices around the turkey breast. Place onto the prepared baking sheet and cover with foil.
3. Bake for 50 minutes. Remove the foil and bake 10 minutes. Pull out baking sheet from oven and set aside for 10 minutes.
4. Cut the turkey breast and serve.

Nutrition

345 Calories

6.5g Fat

56.2g Protein

Turkey Meatloaf

Preparation Time: 15 minutes

Cooking Time: 40 minutes

Servings: 8

Ingredients

Meatloaf

- 2 pounds ground turkey
- 1 cup cheddar cheese
- 1 tablespoon dried onion
- 1 teaspoon dried garlic
- 1 teaspoon garlic powder
- 1 teaspoon red chili powder
- 1 teaspoon ground mustard
- 1 organic egg
- 2 ounces sugar-free BBQ sauce

Topping

- 2 ounces sugar-free BBQ sauce
- 5 cooked bacon slices
- ½ cup cheddar cheese

Directions:

1. Preheat the oven to 400ºF. Grease 9x13-inch casserole dish.
2. For meatloaf:

3. Mix all ingredients. Place into the prepared casserole dish and smooth the surface. Coat the top of meatloaf with BBQ sauce evenly and sprinkle with bacon, then cheese.
4. Bake for 40 minutes. Remove from the oven and set aside. Cut the meatloaf and serve.

Nutrition:

380 Calories

21.7g Fat

40.1g Protein

Herbed Beef Tenderloin

Preparation Time: 15 minutes

Cooking Time: 30 minutes

Servings: 6

Ingredients

- 4 garlic cloves
- ½ cup fresh parsley
- 1/3 cup fresh oregano
- 2 tablespoons fresh thyme
- 2 tablespoons fresh rosemary
- 2 teaspoons fresh lemon zest
- 6 tablespoons olive oil
- 2 tablespoons fresh lemon juice
- ½ teaspoon red pepper flakes
- Salt and ground black pepper
- 1¾ pounds grass-fed beef tenderloin

Directions:

1. Mix all ingredients except for beef tenderloin. Add the beef tenderloin and coat with the herb mixture. Marinate for 45 minutes.
2. Preheat the oven to 425ºF. Remove the beef tenderloin from the bowl and arrange onto a baking sheet. Bake for 30 minutes.

3. Remove the beef tenderloin from oven and place onto a cutting board for 20 minutes. Cut the beef tenderloin and serve.

Nutrition

415 Calories

26.7g Fat

39.2g Protein

Steak with Cheese Sauce

Preparation Time: 15 minutes

Cooking Time: 17 minutes

Servings: 3

Ingredients

Steak

- 2 tablespoons fresh oregano
- ½ tablespoon garlic
- 1 tablespoon fresh lemon peel
- ½ teaspoon red pepper flakes
- Salt and ground black pepper
- 1 (1-pound) (1-inch thick) grass-fed boneless beef top sirloin steak

Cheese Sauce

- 2 tablespoons unsalted butter
- 2 garlic cloves
- 1 tablespoon almond flour
- ½ cup homemade beef broth
- ½ teaspoon dried basil
- ¼ teaspoon dried oregano
- ½ ounce cream cheese
- ¼ cup Parmesan cheese
- ¼ cup heavy cream
- Salt and ground black pepper

Directions:
1. Preheat the gas grill to medium heat. Grease the grill grate. Mix oregano, garlic, lemon peel, red pepper flakes, salt, and black pepper. Rub the steak with garlic mixture.
2. Cook steak onto the grill, covered for 17 minutes.
3. Pull out steak from the grill and set aside for 10 minutes.
4. For cheese sauce:
5. Sauté butter and garlic in the wok over medium heat. Cook flour for about 1 minute. Stir in broth and dried herbs and cook for about 1 minute.
6. Cook in cream cheese, Parmesan cheese and heavy cream for 1 minute. Season and remove from the heat.
7. Cut the steak into desired sized slices and top with cheese sauce. Serve.

Nutrition

461 Calories

25.9g Fat

50.6g Protein

Steak with Pesto

Preparation Time: 10 minutes

Cooking Time: 10 minutes

Servings: 4

Ingredients

- 1 tablespoon butter
- 4 (6-ounce) grass-fed flank steaks
- Salt and ground black pepper
- ½ cup pesto

Directions:

1. Cook the butter in wok over medium-high heat and cook seasoned steaks for 5 minutes per side.
2. Serve with the topping of pesto.

Nutrition

490 Calories

30g Fat

50.4g Protein

Herbed Lamb Chops

Preparation Time: 10 minutes

Cooking Time: 20 minutes

Servings: 4

Ingredients

- 1½ pounds grass-fed lamb loin chops
- 1 tablespoon fresh lemon juice
- ¼ cup fresh parsley
- 2 tablespoons fresh mint leaves
- 1 tablespoon olive oil
- Salt and ground black pepper

Directions:

1. Preheat grill to medium-high heat. Grease the grill grate. Mix lamb loin chops, lemon juice, parsley, mint, oil, salt, and black pepper.
2. Grill for 10 minutes per side. Serve.

Nutrition

350 Calories

16.1g Fat

48g Protein

Stuffed Leg of Lamb

Preparation Time: 20 minutes

Cooking Time: 70 minutes

Servings: 14

Ingredients

- 4 teaspoons olive oil
- ¼ cup scallions
- 2 garlic cloves
- 1 cup fresh spinach leaves
- 2 tablespoons sun-dried tomatoes (in olive oil
- ¼ cup fresh basil leaves
- 2 tablespoons pine nuts
- 2 teaspoons lemon pepper
- ½ cup feta cheese
- 1 (4-5-pound) grass-fed boneless leg of lamb

Directions:

1. Preheat the oven to 325ºF. Greased rack into a roasting pan.
2. Heat 2 teaspoons of olive oil in wok over medium heat and sauté the scallion and garlic.
3. Stir in the spinach, sun-dried tomatoes, basil, pine nuts, and 1 teaspoon of the lemon pepper and cook for 3 minutes.

4. Pull off the heat and stir in feta cheese. Set aside. Remove the strings from leg of lamb and open it. Place the stuffing in the center of meat evenly and roll to seal the filling.
5. Tie the leg of lamb with kitchen string. Coat the rolled leg of lamb with oil and sprinkle with 1 teaspoon of lemon pepper. Arrange the rolled leg of lamb into the prepared roasting pan.
6. Roast for 2 hours. Remove the leg of lamb from the oven and place onto a cutting board.
7. Cover the leg of lamb with foil for 10 minutes before slicing. Serve

340 Calories

15.3g Fat

46.6g Protein

Grilled Pork Chops

Preparation Time: 10 minutes

Cooking Time: 12 minutes

Servings: 4

Ingredients

- ¼ cup fresh basil leaves
- 2 garlic cloves
- 2 tablespoons butter
- 2 tablespoons fresh lemon juice
- Salt and ground black pepper
- 4 (6- to 8-ounce) bone-in pork loin chops

Directions:

1. In a baking dish, mix basil, garlic, butter, lemon juice, salt, and black pepper. Add the chops and coat with the mixture. Cover the baking dish and refrigerate for 45 minutes.
2. Preheat a gas grill to medium-high heat. Grease the grill grate. Cook for 6 minutes per side. Serve.

Nutrition

600 Calories

48g Fat

38.5g Protein

Pork Chops in Cream Sauce

Preparation Time: 15 minutes

Cooking Time: 35 minutes

Servings: 4

Ingredients

- 2 tablespoons olive oil
- 4 large boneless rib pork chops
- Salt
- 3 tablespoons yellow onion
- 2 tablespoons fresh rosemary
- 1/3 cup homemade chicken broth
- 1 tablespoon Dijon mustard
- 1 tablespoon unsalted butter
- 2/3 cup heavy cream
- 2 tablespoons sour cream
- 2 tablespoons fresh parsley

Direction:

1. Cook oil in wok over medium heat and sear the chops with the salt for 4 minutes. Set aside.
2. In the same wok, sauté the mushrooms, onion, and rosemary. Stir in the cooked chops, broth and boil.
3. Select heat to low and cook, covered for 20 minutes. Put aside.

4. In the wok, mix the butter, heavy cream, and sour cream. Stir in the cooked pork chops and cook for 3 minutes. Serve.

Nutrition:

727 Calories

61.4g Fat

39.6g Protein

Garlicky Prime Rib Roast

Preparation Time: 15 minutes

Cooking Time: 75 minutes

Servings: 15

Ingredients

- 10 garlic cloves
- 2 teaspoons dried thyme
- 2 tablespoons olive oil
- 1 (10-pound) grass-fed prime rib roast

Directions:

1. Mix garlic, thyme, oil, salt, and black pepper. Coat the rib roast and arrange in roasting pan, fatty side up. Marinate for 1 hour.
2. Preheat your oven to 500ºF. Roast for 20 minutes. Set temperature to 325ºF and roast for 75 minutes.
3. Remove from the oven and put aside for 15 minutes.

Nutrition:

499 Calories

0.6g Carbs

0.1g Fiber

Beef Wellington

Preparation Time: 20 minutes

Cooking Time: 40 minutes

Servings: 4

Ingredients

- 2 (4-ounce) grass-fed beef tenderloin steaks
- 1 tablespoon butter
- 1 cup mozzarella cheese
- ½ cup almond flour
- 4 tablespoons liver pate

Directions:

1. Preheat your oven to 400°F. Grease a baking sheet. Season.
2. Cook the butter over medium-high heat and sear for 3 minutes per side. Remove from the heat and set aside.
3. Melt the mozzarella cheese in microwave. Sprinkle the almond flour until a dough form. Wrap with parchment paper pieces and roll to flatten it. Remove the upper parchment paper. Divide into 4 pieces.
4. Place 1 tablespoon of pate onto each dough piece and top with 1 steak piece.

5. Cover each steak piece with dough completely. Arrange onto the prepared baking sheet in a single layer. Bake for 30 minutes.

Nutrition:

545 Calories

36.6g I Fat

3g Fiber

Beef with Mushroom Sauce

Preparation Time: 15 minutes

Cooking Time: 28 minutes

Servings: 4

Ingredients

Mushroom Sauce

- 2 tablespoons butter
- 3 garlic cloves
- 1 teaspoon dried thyme
- 1½ cups fresh button mushrooms
- 7 ounces cream cheese
- ½ cup heavy cream

Steak

- 4 (6-ounces) grass-fed beef tenderloin filets
- 2 tablespoons butter

Directions:

1. For mushroom sauce:
2. Sauté garlic, thyme and butter over medium heat
3. Cook seasoned mushrooms for 7 minutes. Lower heat and stir in cream cheese.
4. Cook in cream for 3 minutes.
5. For steak:
6. Season the beef filets

7. In a large cast-iron wok, cook the butter and filets over medium heat for 7 minutes. Pull away from heat and stir in the bacon.
8. Serve with mushroom gravy.

Nutrition:

687 Calories

60g Fat

3.5g Carbs

Herbed Rack of Lamb

Preparation Time: 15 minutes

Cooking Time: 29 minutes

Servings: 8

Ingredients

- 2 (2½-pounds) grass-fed racks lamb
- 2 tablespoons Dijon mustard
- 2 teaspoons fresh rosemary
- 2 teaspoons fresh parsley
- 2 teaspoons fresh thyme

Directions

1. Preheat the charcoal grill to high heat. Grease the grill grate. Season the rack of lamb. Coat the meaty sides of racks with mustard, followed by fresh herbs, press.
2. Situate coals to one side of the grill. Cook racks of lamb over the coals, meaty side down for 6 minutes. Flip the racks and cook for about 3 more minutes.
3. Flip the racks down and move to the cooler side of the grill. Cover and cook for 20 minutes.
4. Remove from the grill and put aside. Serve.

Nutrition

532 Calories

21g Fat
0.4g Fiber

Roasted Leg of Lamb

Preparation Time: 15 minutes

Cooking Time: 75 minutes

Servings: 8

Ingredients

- 1/3 cup fresh parsley
- 4 garlic cloves
- 1 teaspoon fresh lemon zest
- 1 tablespoon ground coriander
- 1 tablespoon ground cumin
- 1 tablespoon smoked paprika
- 1 tablespoon red pepper flakes
- ½ teaspoon ground allspice
- 1/3 cup olive oil
- 1 (5-pound) grass-fed bone-in leg of lamb

Directions:

1. Mix all ingredients (except the leg of lamb).
2. Coat the leg of lamb with marinade mixture.
3. Cover the leg of lamb with plastic and marinate for 8 hours.
4. Remove and keep in room temperature for 30 minutes before roasting.
5. Preheat oven to 350ºF. Arrange the oven rack in the center.

6. Arrange greased rack in the roasting pan.
7. Place the leg of lamb over rack into the roasting pan.
8. Roast for about 1¼-1½ hours, rotating the pan once halfway through.
9. Remove from oven and set aside.
10. Serve.

Nutrition:

610 Calories

29.6g Fat

0.7g Fiber

Baked lamb ribs macadamia with tomato salsa

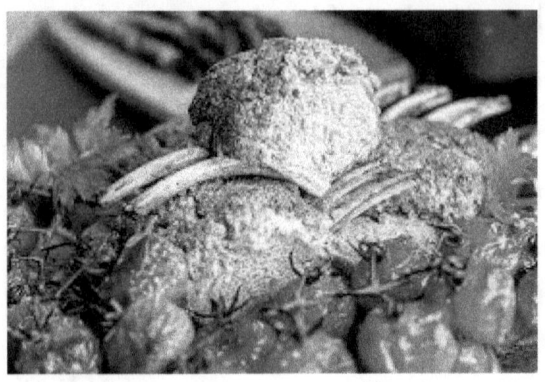

Total time: 45 minutes

Ingredients :

½ pound of fresh lamb ribs

½ cup of cherry tomatoes

½ teaspoon pepper

½ cup of macadamia

½ tablespoon of macadamia oil

¼ cup fresh parsley

1 teaspoon of balsamic vinegar

1 teaspoon of minced garlic

2 tablespoons of extra virgin olive oil

Directions

Cut up the lamb ribs into stripes or pieces

Preheat your oven to 204°C. Ensure that your baking tray is lined with aluminum foil.

Place the macadamia, garlic, parsley, pepper, and olive oil, in the food processor. Blend till the mixture is smooth and lump free.

Rub your processed mixture all over your cut lamb pieces. Ensure that it is coated well enough.

Arrange your strips nicely in the baking tray and bake for 20-25 minutes.

While the lamb bakes, cut the cherry in pieces. You can cut each into four then place them in an aluminum cup.

Pour macadamia oil on the tomatoes. Use spoon to mix the oil and tomatoes without squishing it. The aim is to get the oil all over it.

Take out your lamp and place on a plate.

Place your tomatoes in the over for 4-5 minutes.

Take out the tomatoes and pour sparse amounts of balsamic vinegar and stir.

Pour the tomatoes on the lamb and serve warm.

Grilled Garlic Butter Shrimp

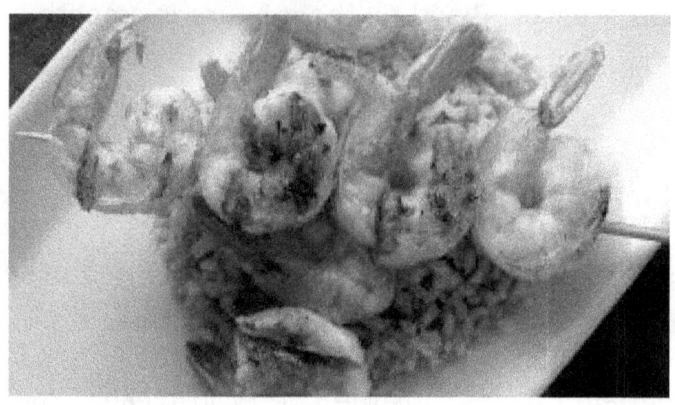

Total time: 35 minutes

Ingredients :

1 pound of large shrimps

1¼ tablespoon of minced garlic

1 teaspoon minced parsley, minced

½ cup of butter

Salt and pepper

Bamboo skewers

Directions

Defreeze, peel, and devein the shrimp. Be careful not to take off the tails.

Preheat the grill to medium heat. This should be around 360°F

Melt your butter.

Mix the melted butter with garlic. Add salt and pepper to your taste.

Put your bamboo skewers through the shrimp

Once grill is heated, place the shrimp on it and start cooking. Turn the shrimp over after 2 minutes.

Spread your garlic and butter mixture on the side facing you.

After two minutes, turn it over and spread the garlic and butter mix on the other side

After you've flipped the shrimp, baste the side facing up with the garlic butter sauce.

Ensure both sides are evenly cooked.

Remove the shrimp and serve

Tomato Chili Chicken Tender with Fresh Basils

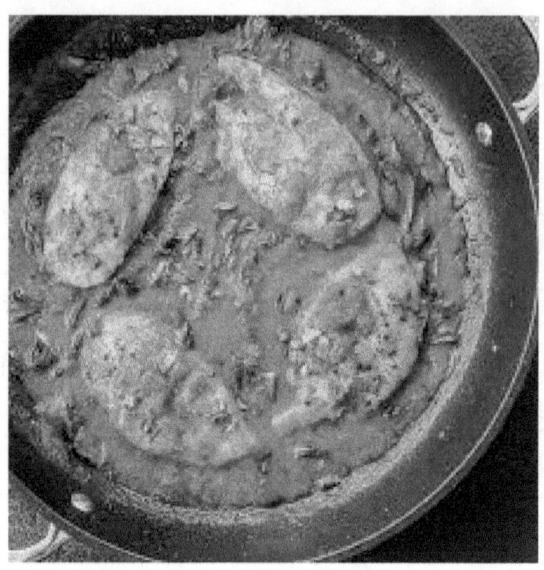

Total time: 50 minutes

Ingredients :

2 pounds of boneless chicken thighs

4 tablespoons extra virgin olive oil

3 lemon grasses

3 tablespoons red chili flakes

2½ tablespoons minced garlic

2 cups water

¼ cup sliced red tomatoes

½ cup fresh basils

Salt and pepper

Directions

Defreeze your chicken

Cut the chicken into small to medium pieces

Place the pieces in a skillet

Add some minced garlic and lemon grass

Add some salt and pepper to taste

Pour water over the chicken

Boil the chicken till the water totally/almost totally evaporates

Take out the chicken and set it aside

Heat a sauce pan and pour olive oil in

Place the chicken and let it cook till it is brown

Place your tomatoes, basils, and chili flakes

Serve warm

Pork crack slaw

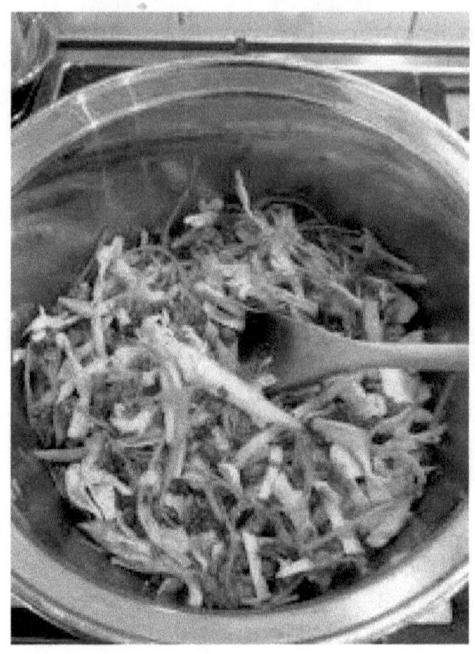

Total time: 30 minutes

Ingredients :

1 pound of ground pork sausage

1 teaspoon of mixed garlic

1 Bags of ready-mix dry coleslaw

1 teaspoon of sesame oil

2 tablespoons of rice vinegar

¼ of a red onion

¼ table spoons of ground ginger

Salt and pepper to taste

Directions

Place the sausage in a bowl and heat till brown and ready, place in chopped red onions while you heat

When the sausage is ready, pour in the rice vinegar, sesame oil, minced garlic, coleslaw kits and salt and pepper to taste.

Stir on fore for five to seven minutes to enable everything cook

Pour in the soy sauce and cover the pot.

Let the contents steam for 5 to ten minutes

While it steams, dice half or a green onion and slice the other half to serve

Take it out and serve warm

Ketogenic lasagna

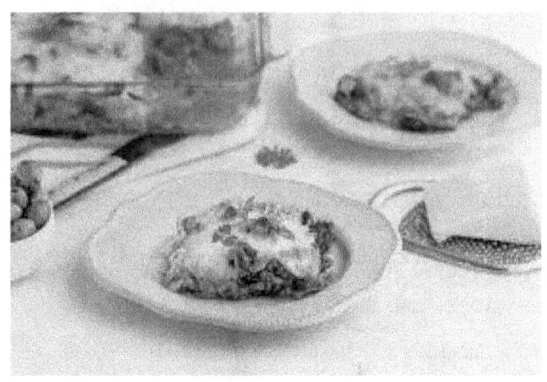

Total time: 30 minutes

Ingredients :

16 ounces of ricotta

8 ounces block cream cheese

4 cups of shredded mozzarella

4 minced cloves of garlic

3 large eggs

2 cups of freshly grated Parmesan cheese

1 tablespoon of extra virgin olive oil

1 ½ table spoons of tomato paste

1 ½ ground beef

¾ cups of marinara

½ white or yellow onion

1 table spoon of dried oregano

Cooking spray, butter, or oil

Pinch crushed red pepper flakes

Chopped parsley

Black pepper

Kosher salt

Directions

Preheat the oven to about 350° F

Lay a cooing parchment or foil on a large baking sheet and grease with cooking oil, or butter.

In another bowl, put in 2 ½ cups of mozzarella, 8 ounces of cheese, and 1 cup of parmesan cheese. Put in all the eggs and mix very well. Add salt and pepper to taste.

Pour on the baking sheet and spread it out

Bake for 15-20 minutes till its golden

Heat some oil in large skillet

Place chopped onion and fry it until it is soft

Add the garlic after and cook for a few more minutes

Poor in tomato paste

Heat the mixture until it is hot enough

Add salt and pepper to taste

Pour in ground beef

Cook the mixture until the meat loses its pink color

Add marinara

Put in red pepper flakes.

Cut noodles in 6 pieces.

Pour in a small amount of the sauce into a baking pan.

Then, put 2 noodles at the base. Divide the ricotta into 3. Spread one part of the ricotta over the broken noodles. Spread another part on the remaining meat and sauce which is on the top. Pour in a last part with the parmesan cheese. Make similar layers and pour cheese at the very top.

Place the mix in the oven until the cheese melts and the sauce heats

Sprinkle parsley and cheese if you wish

Easy meal prep chicken soup

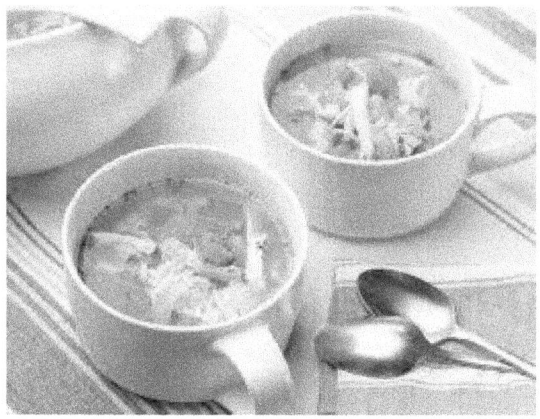

Total time: 45 minutes

Ingredients :

15 chicken breast tenderloins

2 tablespoons garlic powder

1 cup of chopped carrots

1 cup of chopped celery

1 tablespoon butter

Salt

Black pepper

Directions

Unfreeze chicken breast tenderloins

Place in put with 1 ½ cups of water.

Put it a teaspoon of salt

Put in ½ teaspoon of black pepper

Put in 1 tablespoon of garlic

Let the chicken boil for 20-25 minutes till soft and almost ready

Put in chopped carrots and chopped celery

Put in another tablespoon of garlic

Put in butter and cover for 5 to 10 minutes

You can freeze till needed and simply reheat when you need it.

Ketogenic burger

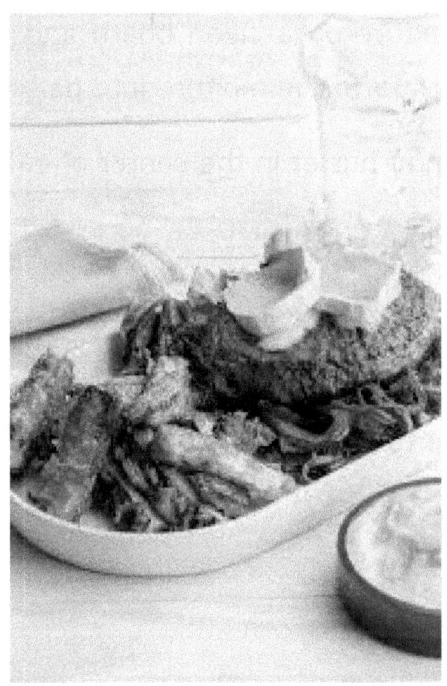

Total time: 50 minutes

Ingredients :

4 pounds of ground hamburger meat

8 tablespoons of half melted butter

5 cloves of garlic, minced

4 tablespoons Worcestershire sauce

1 teaspoon of ground black pepper

1 tablespoon of salt

Directions

Put in the meat, sauce, pepper, and garlic. Put in salt to taste.

Mix the ingredients very well with a big spoon.

Pour out the mixture on a clean board and mold into discs. Use that shape to form the mixture into patties

Put a tablespoon of butter in the center of each patty

Mold the butter into each patty

Place on a grill. Cook each side for around seven minutes

You can try cooking these burgers in foil to prevent it from catching fire due to the increased fat levels

Calamari mayo with cauliflower broccoli salad

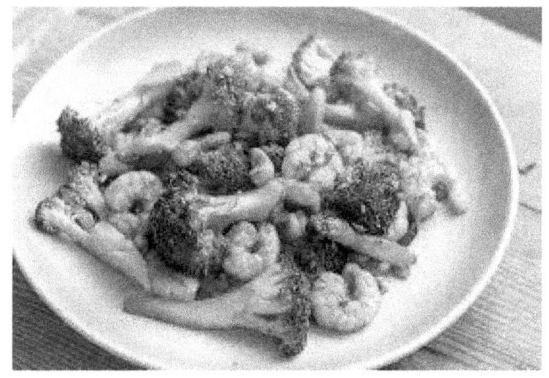

Total time: 35 minutes

Ingredients :

1 ½ pounds of fresh squids

1 ½ tablespoons of lemon juice

2 eggs

2 cups of almond flour

2 cups of broccoli florets

2 cups of cauliflower florets

1 cup of extra virgin olive oil

1 diced onion

½ cup diced cheddar cheese

½ cup of mayonnaise

½ teaspoon of pepper

½ cup of sour cream

Directions

Steam cauliflower and broccoli until they are soft and tender

Place them in bowl for later use

Remove squid ink

Crack eggs

Add salt and pepper to eggs for taste

Cut the squid into rings

Put the squid in the egg mix

Pour in almond flour

Rub in the flour into the squid and egg mix

Heat a pan and pour in oil

Fry the squid in oil until it is golden brown

Take out the squid from the oil and set it aside

In a separate bowl, put in mayonnaise, lemon juice, and sour cream

Mix well

To serve, place the fried squid on a plate with the steam broccoli and cauliflower florets then drip the mayonnaise, lemon juice, and sour cream on it

Sprinkle dry cheddar cheese

Ketogenic strawberry rice

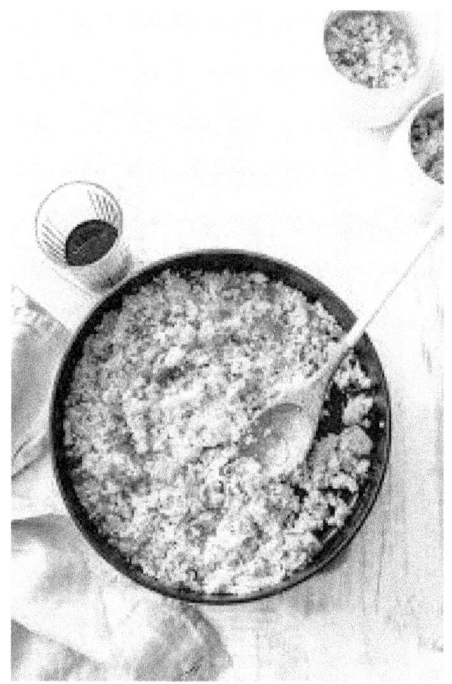

Total time: 40 minutes

Ingredients :

3 cups of sliced strawberries

Cinnamon

2 cup of cooked rice

2 tablespoons of grass-fed butter

2 cup full-fat organic coconut milk

1 tablespoon of pure vanilla extract

½ cup birch xylitol

Himalayan pink salt

¼ teaspoon ground

Directions

Put your 2 ½ cups of sliced strawberries, cinnamon, cooked rice, grass-fed butter, full-fat organic coconut milk, pure vanilla extract, birch xylitol, and a pinch of salt in a saucepan

Cook for 2-30 minutes while stirring till it becomes creamy

Cut up the remaining strawberries

Place the cut up berries on the rice mixture and serve warm

www.ingramcontent.com/pod-product-compliance
Lightning Source LLC
Chambersburg PA
CBHW070722030426
42336CB00013B/1898